Detaching from Sugar

Achieving Emotional and Physical Liberation Through Letting Go

A.T. RAMOS

A.T. RAMOS 1

Contents

A.T. RAMOS

INTRODUCTION

Understanding the Addiction to Sugar

In today's fast-paced environment, sugar has become a staple of our diets, with convenience frequently before nutritious content. Sugar is seductively buried in so many products—from breakfast cereals and snacks to sauces and drinks—that it can be difficult to evade its grip. The basic truth is that sugar consumption has increased over the last few decades, with the average American consuming more than 150 pounds of sugar each year. This surprising statistic highlights a growing sugar addiction as well as a dietary preference that many individuals struggle to understand and ultimately overcome.

Sugar addiction is comparable to chemical dependency since it causes similar molecular reactions in our systems. The brain releases dopamine, a feel-good chemical, in response to sugary treats. It causes sensations of reward and pleasure. This delightful reaction can set off a vicious cycle of cravings, with us returning for more sweets to get the same rush. It's a vicious cycle that frequently leaves us bewildered and unhappy.

Sugar consumption has far more negative consequences for our physical and emotional wellbeing than simply gratifying cravings. Consuming too much sugar has been linked to a variety of health problems, including diabetes, heart disease, obesity, and even certain types of cancer. Furthermore, sugar has a significant impact on our mental health, worsening anxiety, depression, and mood swings. Ironically, the sweets that so many of us rely on for comfort might actually trigger worry. This contradiction represents the basic struggle in our relationship with sugar.

An Overview of Sugar Intake in Contemporary Diets.

To truly understand the magnitude of sugar addiction, we must first consider how we got here. Because processed foods are so widely available, refined sugars and carbohydrates are a staple of modern diets. Our quick meals and instant gratification have become priority for convenience, often at the expense of our health. Sugary foods are not only widely available, but they are also actively promoted and commonly mistaken for healthier options. To compensate for flavor loss, a product branded "low-fat" may contain more sugar, leading consumers to believe they are picking healthier options.

Furthermore, the proliferation of sugary beverages and the rise of fast-food culture have strengthened sugar's grip on our daily lives. Soft drinks, energy drinks, and sweetened coffee have become daily staples for many people, with some drinking them multiple times each day. Our bodies become addicted on sugar as a result of this regular sugar intake, just as they could develop a demand for coffee or nicotine.

Sugar has cultural significance that should not be overlooked, in addition to its convenience in processed foods. Cakes, cookies, and other sweet treats are regularly served to celebrate birthdays, festivals, and other special occasions. Sharing pastries and other sweets with loved ones creates a strong emotional connection to sugar. This is one of the more social elements of dining. Many people discover that sugar has become a vital part of who they are and how they relate with others, so putting it up seems not only terrifying but also lonely.

An explanation of the health and psychological effects of sugar

Knowing how sugar affects our bodies is critical to understanding why letting go of it can lead to considerable freedom. Consuming sugar triggers a cascade of hormonal reactions in the body. Our blood glucose levels rise quickly after ingesting sugar, prompting the pancreas to release insulin. Although insulin is necessary for blood sugar regulation, a high-sugar diet for an extended period of time can lead to insulin resistance, which is the precursor to type 2 diabetes.

Sugar and mental health have a complex relationship. Sugar influences neurotransmitter systems, particularly those involved in mood regulation. Many people experience a brief sugar high followed by a crash, leaving them irritated, fatigued, and with an overwhelming want for more sugar. This trend can result in a chaotic emotional environment in which sugar consumption is closely related with highs and lows.

Furthermore, recent studies have established a link between sugar consumption and an increased risk of anxiety and depression. Consuming much sugar can cause inflammation in the brain, which can lead to mood problems. As we understand more about this relationship, it becomes clear that giving up sugar is a physical, emotional, and psychological process.

The Road Ahead

Setting specific goals and understanding the process's transformative power are critical as you embark on your sugar-free journey. This book seeks to help you understand your relationship with food while also reducing your sugar intake. The purpose of this trip is to liberate yourself physically and emotionally, allowing you to regain control of your body and mind.

Objectives of the Book

Awareness: Being aware is the first step towards liberty. You will learn how to identify the sources of sugar in your diet and how they affect your physical and emotional health as you read this book. You can begin to break the pattern of cravings by identifying your personal triggers.

Education: Knowledge is the way to power. This book will teach you a lot about the science of sugar, its effects on health, and the reasons for our wants. Gaining insight into the core workings of your sugar relationship will allow you to deconstruct it and make the process more manageable.

Practical Strategies: While increasing awareness and educating people is crucial, meaningful change necessitates specific activities. You will discover practical meal planning strategies that promote a sugar-free lifestyle, as well as how to satisfy your sweet tooth in a sugarless way.

Emotional Healing: Releasing yourself from sugar affects your emotional health just as much as your diet. This book will guide you through the emotional aspects of sugar addiction, allowing you to develop better coping methods and a healthier relationship with food.

Community and Support: When you're not alone, it's simpler to make changes. This book emphasizes the importance of creating a support network, whether through friends, family, or internet forums. Resources and tips for connecting with others on similar paths will be available.

How to make the most of this book

To get the most out of this book, approach it with an open mind and a willingness to learn. Here are some tips for making the most of your encounter:

Take Your Time: This is a journey that only you can undertake. Take your time reading the chapters, allowing yourself to assimilate the information and reflect on your experiences.

Interact with the Content: As you read each chapter, take notes in your notebook to record your thoughts, emotions, and developments. Reflecting on your vacation may give insightful views and ideas.

Apply Gradually: Recognize that learning new sugar-reduction approaches will take time. Apply one or two methods at a time, allowing yourself time to make corrections before moving on to the next.

Celebrate your victories, no matter how small. Milestones should be recognized and celebrated. Every step you take to overcome your sugar addiction is a victory and should be applauded.

Seek Assistance: Don't be afraid to seek for help. Having support—whether from friends, family, or online communities—can make the experience less lonely and more enjoyable.

Starting the process of weaning yourself off sweets is a significant self-care action. It's an opportunity to regain control of your health, enhance your mental health, and cultivate a positive connection with food. You are starting the journey of achieving long-term emotional and physical independence by understanding the complexity of sugar addiction and putting the solutions presented in this book to use.

As we move forward, bear in mind that this is a journey about what you stand to gain, not what you are giving up. You will have greater physical and mental stability, as well as healthier interactions with food. Let's take this life-changing trip together, one step at a time.

(Section 1:) (Chapter 1:)

Sugar Science.

Sugar Biology

The Impact of Sugar on the Body and Brain

Sugar, the sweet, crystalline molecule that entices our taste buds and fulfills our cravings, has a tremendous effect on both our bodies and thoughts. When we consume sugar, our cells make glucose, which is their primary source of energy. This seemingly harmless energy source may have a variety of potentially hazardous physiological impacts.

Sugar raises blood glucose levels because it enters the bloodstream fast following ingestion. The pancreas responds by releasing insulin, a hormone necessary for blood sugar regulation. Insulin works like a key, unlocking cells and allowing glucose to enter so it can be used as fuel. However, this is where the story takes a darker turn. Frequent high-sugar consumption can lead to insulin resistance, a condition in which cells lose their capacity to respond to insulin, resulting in elevated blood sugar levels and fat formation. This could lead to serious health issues like type 2 diabetes and obesity.

However, sugar has major harmful effects on both our brains and our bodies. The first glucose rush causes the release of dopamine, a neurotransmitter associated with pleasure and reward. This biological response results in an addictive substance-like dependency cycle. Our brains get increasingly addicted to sugar as we consume more of it, prompting us to seek out our next sugar fix. Understanding this method is critical for people trying to avoid sugar. If we understand the biological basis of these urges, we may be able to confront and ultimately overcome them.

Insulin's role in metabolism

To fully grasp how sugar impacts our bodies, we need to study more about insulin activities and metabolism. Insulin is a vital hormone that controls blood sugar levels as well as how our bodies use and store energy. Sugar consumption raises insulin levels, providing a quick energy boost. However, as blood sugar levels drop, we frequently experience a crash, leaving us exhausted and angry.

The highs and lows that this cycle causes are detrimental to our metabolism. Regular sugar consumption can eventually lead to metabolic dysfunction, which is characterized by excessive blood sugar levels, increased fat storage, and hormonal imbalances. Weight gain, increased hunger, and cravings for more sugary foods are all symptoms of this dysfunction, which contributes to the cycle of sugar addiction.

Furthermore, insulin plays a significant role in fat storage. When we consume more sugar than our bodies require for energy, insulin helps convert the excess glucose to fat, which is then stored as fat in adipose tissue. This mechanism worsens our relationship with sugar by generating weight gain and obesity. Understanding the complicated interplay between sugar, insulin, and metabolism allows us to better prepare for the challenges associated with reducing sugar consumption.

Does Sugar Addiction Exist?

Scientists, medical professionals, and the general public have debated the validity of sugar addiction. Some argue that the biochemical reactions to sugar consumption are similar to those of substance addiction, while others believe it is simply a matter of willpower. According to study, sugar activates the brain's reward circuits in the same way as alcohol and opioids do, causing excessive eating and cravings.

According to research, excessive sugar consumption might cause brain chemical changes similar to those seen in substance addiction. Rats given the option of eating sugar demonstrated indicators of addiction, such as bingeing and withdrawal when the sugar was removed. Although sugar addiction in humans is not as severe as addiction to substances such as cocaine or heroin, the fundamental mechanisms are very similar.

Furthermore, sugar's normalization in society makes it difficult to see it as an addictive chemical. Unlike illegal narcotics, sugar is easily available and socially accepted, making it easy to dismiss the risk of addiction. Because of this cultural foundation, it may be more difficult for people to reduce their sugar consumption because many are unaware of their dependence on it.

Anyone attempting to overcome sugar addiction must recognize that it is a serious issue. By recognizing the powerful pull sugar can have on our bodies and minds, we can begin to design strategies for escape its grip.

(Chapter 2:)

Sugar's Emotional Bond

Using sugar in comfort foods.

When faced with stress or emotional turmoil, many people turn to sweets for solace. It's no surprise that when things get bad, we gravitate toward sweets. Consuming sugar may make us feel snug and nostalgic, transporting us back to simpler, more carefree times. It may be tough to break free from sugar due to this emotional bond, as the comfort it provides can almost seem required.

Our society fosters this link by indulging in sugary treats on holidays and other special occasions such as birthday parties. Sugar has a complex relationship with our memories and emotions, becoming inextricably linked with these sugary joys. Sugar represents joy, happiness, and comfort. However, relying on sugar as a comfort food can lead to unhealthy coping mechanisms, perpetuating the cycle of emotional eating.

To overcome sugar's temptation, one must understand its role as a comfort food. Understanding the emotional triggers that cause us to reach for sugary snacks might help us begin developing healthy coping techniques that do not involve food. This mental change is a necessary first step toward emotional emancipation.

The Impact of Sugar Cravings on the Mind

Sugar cravings have psychological consequences that extend far beyond hunger. When we experience a sugar hunger, our brains communicate a desire for pleasure and reward. This drive may manifest as a strong craving for sweets and is typically accompanied by guilt or shame. Sugar cravings can be powerful, resulting in a vicious cycle of bingeing and guilt trips.

According to research, sweet cravings are associated with emotional dysregulation and mood disorders. When we eat sugar, the brain's reward system is activated, causing us to feel fulfilled and happy. However, this transient high is typically followed by a collapse, leaving us exhausted and irritated. Anxiety and sadness are only two of the psychological issues that this cycle can intensify.

Furthermore, the unfavorable social view linked to sugar consumption may exacerbate feelings of guilt and humiliation. Many people who struggle with sugar cravings may feel isolated and scrutinized, making it even more difficult to break free from these behaviors. Understanding the psychological effects of sugar cravings is vital for cultivating self-compassion and developing healthy routines.

Emotional Eating Cycle

The emotional eating cycle results from the complex interaction of our emotions, behaviors, and food preferences. Stress, grief, and boredom are examples of negative emotions that might cause us to resort to sugar for consolation. Although sugar addiction might give us with temporary reprieve from our feelings, it ultimately leads to a vicious cycle of shame, guilt, and further emotional pain.

To overcome a sugar addiction, it is critical to understand the emotional eating pattern. To change this tendency, we must become more aware of our emotional triggers and develop healthy coping skills. We can look into things that promote emotional well-being, such as exercise, meditation, or creative outlets, instead of seeking sugary snacks.

Furthermore, practicing mindfulness can result in a more pleasant relationship with food. Learning to pay attention to our bodies and emotions allows us to tell the difference between actual hunger and emotional cravings. This understanding allows us to make conscious decisions about what and when to eat, which aids in breaking the cycle of emotional eating.

Finding Added Sugars in Common Foods.

The presence of hidden sugars in ordinary foods is one of the most deceptive aspects of sugar consumption. Many products promoted as "natural" or "healthy" may include a significant amount of sugar, which is sometimes masked behind other labels. Granola bars, yogurt, salad dressings, and sauces are popular offenders because they contain added sugars, increasing our overall consumption.

A.T. RAMOS

Learning to spot hidden sugars is critical for reducing sugar consumption in a healthy way. Knowing the difference between common sugar alternatives such as agave nectar, cane sugar, and high fructose corn syrup will allow you to make more informed grocery purchases. Reduce hidden sugar intake by eating complete, unprocessed foods and carefully reading labels.

It's also critical to understand portion sizes. Given that many boxed meals come in multiple portions, the quantity of sugar in them can quickly add up. Keeping track of portion sizes will help you realize how much sugar you're ingesting and adjust your diet.

Recognize Ingredients and Labels

It can be difficult to read food labels, especially when so many things have a big list of ingredients. However, cutting back on sugar necessitates mastering the art of label reading. Start by paying particular attention to the first few ingredients listed, as they make up the majority of the product. If sugar or a sugar derivative is among the top three ingredients, the product most likely contains a lot of sugar.

Furthermore, be aware of foods labeled as "low sugar" or "sugar-free" because they may contain artificial sweeteners, which carry their own set of health hazards and may not even be the source of the underlying sugar demand. Understanding ingredients and labeling can help you make better selections and reduce the quantity of sugary foods you consume.

Processed Foods' Impact on Sugar Consumption

Processed foods are one of the key drivers of today's increased sugar intake. These meals usually contain added sugars, which may mask the natural flavor of products in order to improve flavor, texture, and shelf life. While processed foods are more convenient, they have a negative impact on our health and well-being.

Because processed meals are so convenient, it is easy to overlook their sugar content. On the other hand, these foods have a significant impact on our health. Consuming substantial amounts of processed sugary meals on a regular basis can lead to metabolic dysfunction, weight gain, and a host of other health issues.

Making a concerted effort to reduce your consumption of processed foods can significantly minimize your sugar intake and improve your overall health. Make an attempt to include entire, unprocessed foods such as fruits, vegetables, whole grains, and lean meats in your diet. This will not only help you consume less sugar, but it will also provide your body with the essential nutrients it requires to maintain overall health.

CALL TO ACTION

Thank you for reading!

I'd like to personally thank you for taking the time to read my work. I really appreciate your time and effort, and I hope this book has provided you with valuable success tools and insights.

Your feedback is really useful to me as I grow as a writer. I would love to hear your feedback, whether positive or negative, so that I may develop and make future works even more useful and fascinating.

I humbly request that you offer an honest evaluation if you found this book worthwhile or if you believe anything may be improved. Your counsel will help me not only improve, but also become a better person.

Thank you again for your support, and I look forward to hearing from you!

A.T. RAMOS

(Section 2:) (Chapter 4:)

Health Effects of Sugar

The Health Effects of Sugar Intake.

Health Risks Associated with Consuming Too Much Sugar

In addition to being a tasty delight, sugar contributes significantly to a growing public health risk. Although it is easy to dismiss the occasional dessert or sugary beverage as a harmless indulgence, the reality is far more concerning. Consuming too much sugar increases the risk of a variety of health issues, many of which are alarmingly common in today's world.

The World Health Organization (WHO) recommends that added sugars comprise no more than 10% of our daily caloric intake. However, many people drink far more than this amount, frequently without even realizing it. The average American consumes over 17 teaspoons of added sugar per day, more than doubling the daily recommended allowance. Overconsumption is related with a variety of health risks, including weight gain, metabolic syndrome, and inflammation.

The effect on weight is one of the most significant topics. Sugar increases calorie consumption while depriving our bodies of essential nutrients. Consuming a lot of sugar can induce an energy imbalance in which our body absorbs more calories than it burns, which can lead to weight gain. This, in turn, provides the conditions for a variety of serious medical problems.

Sugar's Link to Chronic Illnesses (Obesity, Diabetes, Heart Disease)

The link between chronic diseases and excessive sugar consumption is becoming increasingly clear. The most obvious connection is that it is related to type 2 diabetes. A high-sugar diet can cause insulin resistance, a condition in which the body's cells lose sensitivity to insulin. Millions of people worldwide suffer from type 2 diabetes, which is triggered by this resistance. When diabetes develops, the body struggles to control blood sugar levels, triggering a chain reaction of health concerns such as cardiovascular disease, kidney illness, and nerve damage.

In terms of cardiovascular health, sugar's influence on the heart cannot be overlooked. Sugar-rich diets, particularly those high in fructose, have been associated to high blood pressure, triglycerides, and inflammatory markers. These variables influence heart disease, which is one of the leading causes of death around the world. The American Heart Association warns about the link between high sugar consumption and heart disease risk factors, such as fatty liver disease and chronic inflammation.

Obesity, sometimes known as the current pandemic, can result from excessive sugar consumption. Sugary drinks are particularly harmful since they boost calorie intake without making you feel full. These drinks include sodas and sweetened beverages. This may lead to overeating and weight gain. Obesity and sugar consumption have a complicated but apparent relationship: in many populations, obesity prevalence rises in tandem with sugar intake.

Indices of Health Problems Associated with Sugar

Knowing the warning signs of sugar-related health issues is critical for taking control of your health. Unexplained weight gain is one of the most common symptoms of excessive sugar consumption. If you are gaining weight despite following a regular exercise and diet regimen, it may be time to reconsider how much sugar you are consuming.

Fatigue and energy slumps are two other warning signs. Many people experience a crash after the first energy rise caused by sugar, leaving them tired and angry. This vicious cycle may leave you feeling trapped in a cycle of resorting to sugary foods for quick energy spikes, exacerbating pre-existing health issues.

Sugar can also cause a variety of stomach disorders. Eating too much sugar may contribute to bloating, gas, and irregular bowel movements. This is especially true for processed meals, which often contain high-fructose corn syrup.

A.T. RAMOS

Finally, mood fluctuations may indicate sugar-related health concerns. Sugar may be implicated if you notice a significant shift in your emotions or if you feel more worried or depressed than normal. Consuming sugar can disrupt the brain's reward systems, resulting in mood dysregulation and a vicious cycle of cravings and emotional suffering.

Recognizing these warning signals is the first step toward breaking free from sugar's control and regaining your health.

(Chapter 5:)

Emotional and Mental Health.

Sugar's Effects on Mental and Emotional Health

Sugar and mental health have a complex and diverse relationship. Sugar not only provides a quick energy boost, but it also has a significant impact on your mood and emotional wellness. When we eat sugar, our brains release dopamine, which is connected to pleasure and reward. Although this rush of happiness might be rewarding, it is often brief.

When the first high fades, we may experience a "sugar crash" characterized by fatigue, anxiety, and aggravation. Maintaining emotional equilibrium can be challenging when one is on an emotional rollercoaster, which can cause mood instability. Sugar's effects may become less obvious to the brain over time, leading us to need more of it in order to experience the same gratifying feeling. This might lead to a difficult cycle to break.

Furthermore, research suggests that eating a lot of sugar may increase your chances of developing mood disorders such as depression and anxiety. According to some studies, eating too much sugar can induce inflammation in the body, which is increasingly linked to mental health issues. Our bodies may respond to increased sugar consumption by producing systemic inflammation, which can impair cognitive function and emotional regulation.

Sugar's Relationship with Depression and Anxiety

Sugar consumption and mental health are linked in more ways than just mood swings. An accumulating body of research suggests that excessive sugar consumption may contribute to the development of anxiety and depression. This interaction involves complex mechanisms that encompass both psychological and physiological components.

Elevated sugar consumption may cause blood sugar fluctuations, which might trigger anxiety symptoms. These oscillations trigger a vicious cycle of longing, overindulgence, and subsequent collapse, leaving people feeling unsettled and unmanageable. Furthermore, the psychological toll of sugar addiction—the shame and humiliation caused by overindulgence—can exacerbate depressive and anxiety symptoms.

It's worth noting that a higher incidence of depression has been related to the typical Western diet, which is strong in sugar and refined carbs. On the other hand, diets rich in lean proteins, healthy fats, and whole foods have been linked to improved mental health. This relationship stresses the importance of feeding our bodies nutrients that promote mental health while also reducing our sugar intake.

Ways to Boost Emotional Wellbeing Without Sugar

A healthier relationship with food that fosters emotional well-being is essential for breaking free from sugar, rather than simply eliminating sweets from our diets. Without sugar, try these practical strategies to improve your mental well-being:

Mindful Eating: You can improve your connection with food by practicing mindful eating. By taking your time and focusing on the flavors, textures, and fragrances of your meals, you can gain a better appreciation for healthful foods. In addition to minimizing your risk of emotional eating, mindful eating can help you understand your body's hunger and fullness signals.

Investigate New Flavors: If you have a sugar need, consider trying new flavors and meal combinations that will satisfy your hunger without relying on sweets. Adding herbs, spices, and healthy fats might help you feel more pleased with your meals.

Physical Activity: Regular exercise can considerably improve mood and mental health. Endorphins, the body's natural mood boosters, are released during exercise and can help overcome depression and anxiety. On most days of the week, aim for at least 30 minutes of moderate activity.

Seek Support: Surrounding yourself with a supportive group will immensely improve your journey to overcome your sugar addiction. Joining a support group or approaching friends and family who are aware of your goals can be beneficial. Sharing your experiences and struggles may assist to foster a sense of accountability and connection.

Practice Stress Reduction: Stress is a common trigger for sugar cravings. Learning healthy stress coping strategies like yoga, deep breathing techniques, or meditation might help you deal with emotional triggers more effectively. Developing alternative coping methods for stress and weariness will reduce the need for sweets to provide relief.

Emphasis on Nutrient-Dense Foods: Give your body and mind the nourishment they require by prioritizing whole, nutrient-dense foods. Omega-3 fatty acid-rich meals, such as nuts, seeds, and fatty fish, have been linked to improved mood and cognitive function. A diet rich in fruits, vegetables, and whole grains can also provide essential vitamins and minerals for emotional health.

Implementing these approaches can help you achieve emotional well-being that is not dependent on sugar. Even if it takes some time, each action you take will bring you one step closer to a better, more balanced lifestyle.

(Section 3:) (Chapter 6:)

The Let Go Process

Understanding Your Sugar Reactions

Finding Your Personal Sugar Craving Triggers

Giving up sugar entails more than just eliminating sweets from your diet; it involves a deep dive into self-awareness. Finding out what causes your sugar addiction is one of the first steps in this process. Triggers are the specific conditions, sensations, or surroundings that cause you to crave sweets. It's critical to recognize them so that you may devise strategies for effectively regulating those wants.

Common triggers include stress, boredom, social occasions, and even certain times of day when you're more likely to need something sweet. Do you crave sugar after a difficult day at work or when relaxing on the couch? The first step toward breaking the emotional eating cycle is recognizing these tendencies.

To start identifying your triggers, consider your most recent sugar cravings. Consider the following questions for yourself.

When do I crave sweets the most?
What emotions arise for me when I experience these cravings?

Are there any specific settings or circumstances that promote me to overeat sweet foods?

What is my regular response when I have these cravings?

You can prepare to react differently when these triggers appear by being aware of them and shifting your focus from mindless consumption to thoughtful decision-making.

Keep a Dietary Record for Awareness

A food journal is one of the most useful tools for this operation. Keeping a food and feelings journal can teach you a lot about your emotional responses and sugar consumption patterns. Keeping a food journal encourages attention and allows you to discover how you're eating habits and mood are related.

Here's how to maintain a productive food journal:

Be Reliable: Every day, record your meals in your food notebook. Keep a log of everything you eat and drink, including the time of day and how you felt while eating. Patterns can be recognized throughout time based on consistency.

Examine Your Entries: At the end of each week, review your entries. Keep an eye out for recurring patterns or triggers, such as certain feelings or situations that cause you to crave sugar. Understanding these relationships allows you to design future approaches to them.

Celebrate Your Achievements: Don't forget to express gratitude for the wise choices you've made along the road. Celebrate your victory if you were able to avoid reaching for sugar while navigating a trigger! Acknowledging your progress promotes positive behavior and boosts drive.

Make Use of Technology: Consider using smartphone apps designed for tracking food. You may enter emotions into many of these tools, making it easier to investigate how your emotions influence you're eating habits.

A food diary can help you build self-awareness, which is essential for long-term transformation, as well as serving as a tracking tool.

Mindfulness techniques for overcoming cravings

You may take back control of your sugar cravings with the help of mindfulness, which is a very useful technique. Practicing mindfulness allows you to learn to see your urges objectively and respond to them with intention rather than impulsiveness. You can integrate the following mindfulness practices into your regular routine:

Breathing exercises: Pause for a second if you feel a sugar craving coming on. Pay attention to how you breathe. Breathe deeply through your nose for four counts, hold for four counts, and then slowly exhale through your mouth for six counts. Do this multiple times. This simple pastime can help you relax and reduce the intensity of your appetite.

Perform a body scan exercise to connect with your physical sensations. Close your eyes, find a comfortable place to sit or lie down, and focus on each part of your body, starting with your toes and progressing to the top of your head. Take note of any sore spots or areas of tension. By developing self-awareness, you can lessen your proclivity to go for sugar when you're sad.

When you do indulge in a pleasure, remember to eat attentively. Take your time and appreciate each bite. Take note of the aromas, flavors, and textures. This strategy can help you feel less reliant on added sugar by improving your dining experience and training you to appreciate food more.

Make time each day to express gratitude. Think of three things for which you are grateful every day. By shifting your focus from desires to appreciation, you can improve your emotional fortitude and reduce your need to turn to sugar for comfort.

By practicing mindfulness, you offer yourself the ability to firmly and clearly manage cravings, making it easier to overcome your sugar addiction.

(Chapter 7:)

How To Live Without Sugar

How to Reduce Sugar Consumption Gradually.

The transition to a sugar-free lifestyle does not have to be a one-way street. Actually, gradually reducing sugar consumption is easier to maintain and more sustainable. This extensive guide will help you gently move to a sugar-free diet.

Establish Achievable Objectives: Begin by defining self-achievable goals. Instead of completely eliminating sugar, try to reduce it by a certain percentage over the course of a few weeks. This will help you avoid feeling overwhelmed if you tackle the task gradually.

Determine Your Sources: Consider how much sugar you now consume. Examine your food journal to discover where sugar may be creeping into your diet. This could include processed foods, sugary drinks, and snacks or desserts. Knowing where your sugar comes from will help you focus on gradually reducing or eliminating it.

Pick Your Battles: There are distinctions between sugar sources. Prioritize reducing processed foods and added sugars before tackling the naturally occurring sugars found in fruits. This allows you to continue getting the benefits of whole fruits while also supporting you in making noticeable progress.

Replace One Item at a Time: Instead of attempting to eliminate all sugar from your diet at once, replace one sugar-containing item each week with a healthier one. Try substituting your morning sugary cereal with oatmeal topped with nuts and fresh fruit, for example. Your taste buds can adapt to this incremental technique without feeling deprived.

Plan for Difficulties: Identify potential hurdles and devise strategies to overcome them. For example, if you tend to have sugar cravings after dinner, prepare healthier dessert options or find something entertaining to do while you're busy.

Follow Your Development: Celebrate every small victory you achieve along the way. To track your progress, use an app or keep a notepad. Acknowledging your victories, no matter how modest, can boost motivation and encourage positive behavior.

Sugar substitutes include natural sweeteners and nutritious snacks.

It's critical to find acceptable substitutes as you cut back on sugar. Fortunately, you may still eat a balanced diet without adding sugar owing to a selection of natural sweeteners and nutritious snacks.

Natural Sweeteners: Instead of refined sugar, consider using natural sweeteners. Sweetening alternatives such as agave nectar, stevia, maple syrup, and honey can be used without having the same negative health consequences as refined sugars. Remember that even when using natural sweeteners, moderation is key!

Healthy Snacks: Stock up on nutritious snacks to satisfy hunger and energize your body. Nuts, yogurt, fresh fruits, and vegetables with hummus are excellent choices. Energy balls made with oats, nut butter, and natural sweeteners are a hearty treat.

Try Different Flavors: Look for ways to enhance the flavor of your food without adding sugar by using herbs and spices. Herbs such as basil and mint can enhance savory dishes, whilst nutmeg, cinnamon, and vanilla extract can add delicious sweetness to cuisine.

Emphasis on Whole Foods: Refocus your attention on whole foods that nourish your body. Incorporate plenty of fruits, veggies, whole grains, lean meats, and healthy fats into your meals. In addition to supporting physical health, a nutrient-dense diet can help regulate your mood and reduce your craving for sweets.

Meal Planning and Preparation Tips: Planning your snacks and meals ahead of time will allow you to avoid making quick decisions when cravings strike. Create a weekly eating plan that includes nutritious snacks and balanced meals. Preparing and preparing items in bulk can help you stick to your sugar-free lifestyle.

(Chapter 8:)

Building a Network of Support

The Value of Support and Community

You do not have to start the process of reducing your sugar consumption on your own. In reality, one of the most significant aspects of establishing a long-term sugar-free lifestyle is forming a support network. As you work toward your goals, a community of like-minded individuals may provide accountability, motivation, and support.

Friends, relatives, coworkers, and internet communities, among others, can provide assistance. Sharing your goals with others fosters a sense of community by inviting them to go with you.

Locating Groups or Partners for Accountability

The advantages of having an accountability partner can be immense. This could be a friend or family member who shares your goals and wants to cut back on sugar consumption. Frequent check-ins allow you to celebrate accomplishments, discuss challenges, and support one another, all of which can help you stay committed and focused.

Consider forming or joining a support group for healthy eating and lifestyle changes in your town or online. These communities routinely share advice, how-tos, and success stories to inspire and motivate you. Interacting with people who share similar goals may make the journey feel less lonely and more enjoyable.

Resources (websites, forums, apps) for ongoing assistance

A variety of resources are available to help you establish a sugar-free lifestyle. These resources, ranging from websites and forums to apps, can provide ongoing guidance and inspiration.

Apps: Consider using apps that help you track your food intake, give recipes, and connect you to useful networks. Using applications like MyFitnessPal, Chronometer, and Noom can help you track your progress and make informed decisions.

Check out websites and blogs that promote wellness, sugar reduction, and healthy eating. Many of them include useful resources such as meal planning, recipes, and professional guidance. Another alternative is to be motivated by health-conscious influencers.

Online Forums: Join social media groups and online forums dedicated to sugar reduction and healthy living. Interacting with others in these forums allows you to ask questions, share experiences, and learn from individuals who have conquered similar problems.

(Section 4:) (Chapter 9:)

Accepting Emancipation.

The Benefits of Giving Up.

The Health and Mental Benefits of Giving Up Sugar

Giving up sugar is more than just a dietary change; it is a call to embrace a new, exciting way of life. Adopting a sugar-free diet provides numerous substantial and far-reaching benefits for both physical and mental health.

1. Enhanced Well-being

Reducing sugar consumption has various immediate advantages, one of which is better physical health. High sugar intake has been linked to a variety of health concerns, including heart disease, diabetes, and obesity. Many people find that reducing their sugar intake leads to weight loss, increased energy, and improved metabolic health.

Weight management: Cutting less on sugar helps control appetite and reduces the desire for unhealthy foods. This change may result in long-term weight loss, lowering the risk of obesity-related ailments. When sugary foods are eliminated from their diets, many people find that they naturally gravitate towards more nutrient-dense options and no longer need to count calories.

Blood Sugar Stability: One of the most significant advantages of cutting off sweets is improved blood sugar control. People with type 2 diabetes or insulin resistance may benefit from a sugar-free diet since it helps stabilize blood glucose levels and reduces the danger of spikes and crashes. This regularity may result in fewer cravings and higher energy levels throughout the day.

Heart Health: Excess sugar consumption is linked to excessive triglycerides, high blood pressure, and inflammation, all of which are risk factors for heart disease. Cutting down on sugar can improve your cardiovascular health and lower your risk of heart attacks and strokes.

2. Improved mood and mental clarity.

Eliminating sugar has numerous physical benefits, but it can also significantly enhance mental and emotional health. Many people report that giving up sugar has improved their concentration, reduced anxiety, and improved mood stability.

Mood Regulation: Sugar can trigger mood changes similar to those seen on roller coasters. Eating sugary foods frequently results in an initial energy rush followed by a collapse that may leave you feeling irritated or exhausted. Your blood sugar can be controlled, allowing you to have more consistent energy and a better mood all day.

Decreased Anxiety and Depression: There appears to be a clear link between eating and mental health. Consuming substantial amounts of sugar has been related to an increased risk of sorrow and anxiety. Adopting a sugar-free diet may improve your general health and reduce the symptoms of certain diseases.

Mental Clarity: Many people report that cutting back on sugar improves their concentration and cognitive performance. When the brain is not reliant on sugar for energy, it may function more effectively, producing improved thinking and productivity.

Success Stories: Real Changes in People's Lives

Adopting a sugar-free lifestyle can be difficult, but many individuals have done so and seen wonderful results. Their stories are a powerful source of inspiration for anyone thinking about giving up sweets.

1. Maria's Trip

Maria, a 35-year-old mother of two, has spent years suffering with fatigue and weight fluctuations. She decided to eliminate additional sugars from her diet after finding that there was a link between sugar consumption and health problems. Maria lost thirty pounds in a matter of months and had significant improvements in her mood and energy levels. She elaborates: "I never realized how much sugar was depressing me." "I felt lighter, both mentally and physically, after letting go of it."

2. David's transformation

David, a fifty-year-old accountant, has been dealing with type 2 diabetes for almost ten years. He chose to eliminate sugar from his diet after hearing a health lecture that highlighted its dangers. His blood sugar levels recovered to normal in six months, and he was able to reduce his medication significantly. According to David, "it was like flipping a switch." I not only lost weight, but also reclaimed my life. I feel like I'm back in my 30s!"

3. Jennifer Takes Charge

Jennifer, a 28-year-old graphic designer, discovered that her cravings for sweet treats often corresponded with times of stress. After making the decision to take charge, she gave up sugar and focused on whole foods. The result was a decrease in her anxiety and an increase in her energy. "I've discovered healthier ways to manage stress," she says. "Now, instead of reaching for sugar, I reach for a good book."

Honoring Achievement and Advancement
Commencing a sugar-free lifestyle necessitates celebrating your triumphs and advancements; every step you take is a success, and recognizing these gains keeps you motivated to maintain your health.

Establish Milestones: Set clear, attainable objectives for yourself. Setting goals helps you keep motivated and focused. Examples of these goals include cutting back on sugar by a certain percentage, giving up sugar-filled beverages, or going a week without ingesting any added sugar.

Record Your Journey: Keep track of your progress using an app or a notebook, and write about the mental and physical changes you experience. This type of introspection can be a powerful source of motivation when times are tough.

Celebrate Small Victories: No matter how small your win may be, it should be acknowledged and celebrated. By rewarding yourself with a new gym outfit, a stress-relieving spa day, or simply indulging in a favorite nutritious meal, you may reinforce your commitment to living a sugar-free lifestyle.

Tell Your Story: By sharing your story with friends, family, or online communities, you might inspire others and strengthen your own commitment. You never know who might benefit from your knowledge and experiences!

(Chapter 10:)

Long-term Success Strategies

maintaining an abstinence-based lifestyle

Maintaining your commitment to a sugar-free lifestyle over time is critical after you've embarked on it. Long-term change necessitates sustainability, and there are several strategies you may employ to ensure it occurs.

1. Continue Your Education: Stay up to date on nutrition and the harmful health consequences of sugar by reading books, listening to podcasts, and following experts in the field. The more you learn about sugar's effects, the more motivated you will be to avoid it.

2. Meal planning: Setting aside a few hours each week to plan and prepare your meals can make it easier to stick to your sugar-free goals. When hunger strikes, eating nutritious meals and snacks ahead of time reduces the temptation to reach for sugary convenience foods.

3. Mindful Eating Practices: Make mindful eating a part of your daily life by savoring each bite of food, paying attention to the flavors and textures, and paying attention to your hunger cues. Mindful eating not only promotes a better relationship with food, but it can also reduce mindless snacking.

4. Find Healthier Substitutes: Keep healthful substitutes for sugary foods in your cabinet. Stock up on wholegrain snacks, nuts and seeds, and fresh fruits. Swapping out sweet goods for healthier alternatives can make you less likely to reach for sugar when cravings occur.

Handling Obstacles and Failures

Setbacks are unavoidable on any path to advancement; it is vital to acknowledge this and plan ahead of time on how to deal with them.

1. Develop Self-Compassion: If you find yourself giving in to cravings or overindulging in sugar, work on your self-compassion. Instead of criticizing yourself, accept that mistakes are unavoidable during the process, refocus on your goals, and learn from the experience rather than wallowing in guilt.

2. Determine Triggers: Take advantage of setbacks to pinpoint probable causes. Consider the circumstances that preceded your cravings and how you might deal with those triggers differently in the future. Gaining a more profound understanding of your habits will allow you to overcome obstacles with greater efficiency.

3. Seek Support: In times of need, don't be afraid to seek for help. Having a support system, whether it's talking to friends, joining an online support group, or consulting a medical specialist, can help you stay motivated and accountable.

4. Reframe and Reflect: When faced with difficulties, pause to contemplate your route. Remind yourself of your accomplishments and why you chose to give up sweets. Rethinking failures as opportunities for progress may help you maintain an optimistic outlook.

Developing a Positive Connection with Food

Making the switch to a sugar-free diet means more than just eliminating sugar; it also entails developing a healthier relationship with food, which may have a long-term impact on your health.

1. Prioritize whole, nutrient-dense foods rich in vitamins and minerals. Instead of viewing food as a source of guilt, view it as a means of nourishing your body and promoting good health.

2. Embrace Variety: To keep your meals interesting, experiment with new cuisines and flavors. Trying new dishes and ingredients can renew your passion of cooking while also adding fun to eating healthily.

3. Following Intuitive Eating Principles: By paying attention to your body's signals of hunger and fullness, you may cultivate a flexible, balanced relationship with food and indulge in sweets guilt-free on occasion.

4. Celebrate All Foods: Rather than categorizing foods as "good" or "bad," emphasize moderation and balance. You should be able to enjoy a wide range of foods, including those that are not considered "healthy." This mental shift can reduce cravings and promote a healthier relationship with food.

Final Thoughts: Examining The Experience

As we near the end of our investigation into the significant effects of sugar on our lives and the powerful process of letting go, it's important to reflect on our shared journey. This journey is about breaking free from the limitations that sugar has placed on our emotional stability, physical well-being, and connection to food—it's not just about eliminating one item from our diets.

Highlighting Critical Findings

Throughout this book, we have thoroughly examined the various aspects of sugar consumption and its effects. We have illustrated the difficulties presented by sugar in a clear and concise manner, detailing the physiological effects of high sugar consumption as well as its link to long-term conditions such as diabetes, heart disease, and obesity. The following are some of the most noteworthy points:

1. Identifying Sugar's Physical Effects

We started our journey by realizing the observable health hazards related to sugar consumption. We talked about how consuming too much sugar can raise insulin resistance, cause significant weight gain, and increase the chance of developing chronic illnesses. This knowledge should act as a wake-up call, motivating us to choose the meals we eat carefully. Adopting a sugar-free diet can reap a host of health benefits, such as increased energy, better weight control,

2. Accepting Your Emotional Well-Being

In addition to being a source of energy, sugar consumption has been linked to mental health issues such as anxiety and depression, prompting us to look for healthier ways to manage our emotions. The psychological and emotional aspects of sugar consumption were also investigated, and it became clear that sugar had a significant influence on our mood, anxiety levels, and general mental health. By replacing sugar with nutritious foods, we can create an emotional

3. The Impact of Mindfulness and Awareness.

Throughout the book, we emphasized the importance of identifying our sugar triggers and practicing mindfulness to combat cravings. Understanding our relationship with food necessitates taking important actions such as keeping a food diary, engaging in mindfulness exercises, and recognizing our emotional eating patterns. This understanding not only allows us to make better decisions, but it also increases our capacity for self-compassion as we go through life.

4. How to Lead a Sugar-Free and Sustainable Lifestyle

We outlined doable strategies for adopting a sugar-free lifestyle, including meal planning, locating healthy substitutes, and gradually cutting back on sugar consumption. All of these tactics serve to bolster the notion that long-term transformation is both feasible and achievable. It is about adopting a holistic approach to eating that prioritizes health and well-being over simply cutting out sugar.

5. Creating a Network of Support

One of the most profound realizations we had along this path was the importance of support and community; meeting like-minded people, forming support networks, and finding accountability partners can all provide priceless inspiration and drive. A sense of belonging fosters resilience, making it easier to overcome obstacles and share in victories.

6. Long-Term Success Strategies

Finally, we discussed long-term strategies for adhering to a sugar-free diet, emphasizing the importance of continuous learning, self-compassion, and developing a positive relationship with food. By adopting intuitive eating concepts and shifting our perspective from restriction to nourishment, we can cultivate a healthy relationship with food that will benefit us for many years to come.

Motivation for Continued Development and Emancipation

As you finish this book, I'd like to leave you with a word of encouragement: sugar-free living is a highly personal journey with many ups and downs; it requires perseverance, dedication, and an openness to change. However, keep in mind that the goal of this journey is to regain your health, vitality, and sense of joy in life—not just to give up sweets.

1. Recognize your advancement.

Consider your personal journey and celebrate your accomplishments, whether you are just starting out or have already made significant changes in your life to reduce sugar. Celebrate the small victories, such as the times you chose a nutritious snack over a sugary treat, or the times you recognized a craving and decided to act sensibly in response. Every step you take demonstrates your strength and determination.

2. Accept the process of learning.

Recognize that learning is a constant on this trip. Along the journey, there may be obstacles, temptations, and disappointments, but every event presents an opportunity for development. Accept these experiences as worthwhile lessons that will guide your decisions going forward. You'll get better at negotiating the nuances of cravings and emotional triggers as you learn more about your body and your relationship with food.

3. Develop a Growth Attitude.

Developing a growth mindset is essential for long-term success. Take a curious, rather than judgmental, approach to your journey, viewing obstacles as stepping stones toward a deeper understanding of who you are and what you need, rather than as failures. This perspective allows you to recover from setbacks, change, and develop.

4. Make self-care and wellbeing a top priority.

While adjusting to a sugar-free lifestyle, prioritize your well-being and self-care. Consume nutritious foods, exercise regularly, and practice mindfulness and relaxation. These habits will strengthen your resolve to live a sugar-free life while also improving your overall health.

5. Tell us your story.

By sharing your experiences on social media, blogging, or in one-on-one interactions, you can encourage and inspire others to embark on their own journeys toward emancipation. By sharing your struggles and insights, you can create a supportive and encouraging group that spreads positive change.

6. Stay Aware of Your Why

Finally, remember your "why." Consider the reasons you chose to give up sweets and live a healthier lifestyle; your motivations can help guide your decisions and keep your commitment, whether it's to improve your health, lift your mood, or set a good example for loved ones.

A Prospective Perspective.

Accept the journey as an ongoing process of growth that invites you to experiment with new eating, sleeping, and emotional patterns. As you move forward, imagine yourself energized, free of cravings, and ready to make decisions that support your health goals.

Finally, keep in mind that giving up sugar is a meaningful gift you give to yourself. It's a call to embrace life to the fullest, relish each second, and develop a profound sense of wellbeing. Although the journey may be difficult, the benefits are immense. Watch as your life changes in stunning, unexpected ways as you welcome this adventure with open arms and a heart full of love.

Cheers to your well-being, joy, and emancipatory adventure!

CALL TO ACTION

Thank you for reading!

I'd like to personally thank you for taking the time to read my work. I really appreciate your time and effort, and I hope this book has provided you with valuable success tools and insights.

Your feedback is really useful to me as I grow as a writer. I would love to hear your feedback, whether positive or negative, so that I may develop and make future works even more useful and fascinating.

I humbly request that you offer an honest evaluation if you found this book worthwhile or if you believe anything may be improved. Your counsel will help me not only improve, but also become a better person.

Thank you again for your support, and I look forward to hearing from you!

A.T. RAMOS